WORLD HEALTH ORGANIZATION

INTERNATIONAL AGENCY FOR RESEARCH ON CANCER

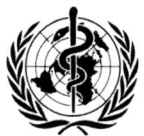

IARC
Working Group Reports
Volume 4

# IARC CODE OF GOOD SCIENTIFIC PRACTICE

This report represents the views and expert opinions of an
IARC Working Group that met in Lyon, France

4-5 May 2006,
16-17 November 2006
and 26 June 2008

Published by the International Agency for Research on Cancer,
150 cours Albert Thomas, 69372 Lyon Cedex 08, France

© International Agency for Research on Cancer, 2008

Distributed by
WHO Press, World Health Organization, 20 Avenue Appia, 1211 Geneva 27, Switzerland
(tel: +41 22 791 3264; fax: +41 22 791 4857; email: bookorders@who.int).

Publications of the World Health Organization enjoy copyright protection in accordance with the provisions of Protocol 2 of the Universal Copyright Convention. All rights reserved.

The designations employed and the presentation of the material in this publication do not imply the expression of any opinion whatsoever on the part of the Secretariat of the World Health Organization concerning the legal status of any country, territory, city, or area or of its authorities, or concerning the delimitation of its frontiers or boundaries.

The mention of specific companies or of certain manufacturers' products does not imply that they are endorsed or recommended by the World Health Organization in preference to others of a similar nature that are not mentioned. Errors and omissions excepted, the names of proprietary products are distinguished by initial capital letters.

The authors alone are responsible for the views expressed in this publication.

The International Agency for Research on Cancer welcomes requests for permission to reproduce or translate its publications, in part or in full. Requests for permission to reproduce or translate IARC publications – whether for sale or for noncommercial distribution – should be addressed to WHO Press, at the above address (fax: +41 22 791 4806; email: permissions@who.int).


**IARC Library Cataloguing in Publication Data**

IARC code of good scientific practice / IARC Working Group on Scientific Practice

    (IARC Working Group Reports ; 4)

    1. Biomedical Research – standards  2. Ethics, Research  3. Research Design
    I. IARC Working Group on Scientific Practice  II. Series

    ISBN 978-92-832-2445-7                     (NLM Classification:  W 20.5)

# LIST OF PARTICIPANTS

**Dr Philippe Autier**
IARC
150, cours Albert Thomas
69008 Lyon

**Dr Paolo Boffetta**
IARC
150, cours Albert Thomas
69008 Lyon

**Dr Peter Boyle**
IARC
150, cours Albert Thomas
69008 Lyon

**Dr Paul Brennan**
IARC
150, cours Albert Thomas
69008 Lyon

**Dr Silvia Franceschi**
IARC
150, cours Albert Thomas
69008 Lyon

**Professor Charles Gillis**
Glasgow, UK

**Mrs Caroline Granger**
IARC
150, cours Albert Thomas
69008 Lyon

**Professor Adele Green**
Queensland Institute of Medical Research
Brisbane 4029, Queensland
Australia

**Dr Pierre Hainaut**
IARC
150, cours Albert Thomas
69008 Lyon

**Dr Fabio Levi**
Registre vaudois des Tumeurs
Institut universitaire de Médecine Sociale et Préventive
CHUV – Falaises 1
1011 Lausanne
Switzerland

**Lord Mackay of Clashfern**
Inverness, UK

**Dr David McNamee**
The Lancet
32 Jamestown Road
London NW1 7BY
UK

**Dr Berit Mørland**
The Norwegian Health Services Research Centre
St Olavs Plass
0130 Oslo
Norway

**Dr Hiroko Ohgaki**
IARC
150, cours Albert Thomas
69008 Lyon

**Dr Tikki Pang**
WHO
Avenue Appia 20
1211 Geneva 27
Switzerland

**Mr Markus Pasterk**
IARC
150, cours Albert Thomas
69008 Lyon

**Professor You-Lin Qiao**
Cancer Institute Beijing
17 South Panjiayuan Lane
Beijing 100021
People's Republic of China

**Dr Hans Storm**
Danish Cancer Society
Strandboulevarden 49
DK-2100 Copenhagen
Denmark

**Dr Sean Tavtigian**
IARC
150, cours Albert Thomas
69008 Lyon

**Dr Alexander Walker**
WHISCON
P.O. Box 775
Westwood, MA 02090
USA

# Foreword

Every Institute which does research is potentially vulnerable to a number of issues ranging across a wide spectrum from poor study logistics to flagrant misconduct by any individual on its faculty. IARC may be potentially more vulnerable given the frequent international, multicentric nature of its study data collection. With the increasing globalisation of the IARC research programme, it is imperative to ensure the same level of protection of study subjects irrespective of the geographical and social location of the study. This is a key focus for the newly-established IARC Ethics Committees (Institutional Review Board and Ethics Review Committee).

In addition, the extensive international collaborations that IARC has in their studies also offers increased risk of poor quality data, arising from a variety of reasons ranging from accidental errors to outright scientific fraud. The increasing incorporation of biological measurements in all IARC epidemiological studies increases further the need for care and vigilance.

In all, it is essential to work with the broad Scientific Community and the IARC Ethics Committees to develop guidelines for the development, conduct, analysis and publication of all IARC studies. The work to be done for the IARC studies would also be applicable internationally to other groups and the development of guidelines would also benefit from international input and involvement.

Accordingly, in March 2005, the IARC Cabinet approved the development of a Code of Good Scientific Practice for IARC faculty and collaborators and created an external committee with the charge to prepare such a Code. Thus, an IARC Working Group was established to develop a *Code of Good Practice for IARC Research Studies*. Issues to be addressed include study design, ethics approval, informed consent, study conduct, avoidance of errors (accidental or deliberate), data audit, peer review and publication.

An initial draft Code of Good Scientific Practice was developed and then this was used in the field for one year. After this year, comments received about the Code of Good Scientific Practice were considered by the Working Group and the resultant final version is contained in the following pages.

It is a pleasure to acknowledge and thank the membership of the Working Group for their diligence and skill in helping in this important initiative for IARC. The resultant Code is available for all the scientific community to consider and to use.

**Peter Boyle PhD**
**Director**

# IARC's Mission

The objective of the International Agency for Research on Cancer is to promote international collaboration in cancer research with the objective of improving health through a reduction in the incidence of and mortality from cancer throughout the world.

The Agency makes provision for planning, promoting and developing research in all phases of the causation, treatment and prevention of cancer; for collection and dissemination of information on the epidemiology of cancer, on cancer research and on the causation and prevention of cancer throughout the world; for studies on the natural history of cancer; and for education and training of personnel for research on cancer.

IARC's mission is to accomplish the work outlined in the Statute to the highest standards possible, both scientific and ethical; to become the leading international centre in research for cancer prevention and provide leadership to the international community engaged in research in cancer prevention and control world-wide.

# Preamble

The IARC Code of Good Scientific Practice is intended to guide research conducted within IARC premises, and to be embedded in its relationships with others. It will also apply to the Working Groups composed of external experts and convened by IARC. The code complements the IARC Guidelines on Ethics; all research programmes are subject to prior approval by the IARC Institutional Review Board and the IARC Ethics Review Committee, other institutional or national Ethics Review Boards as required. Any deviation from the Code of Good Scientific Practice must be justified.

Rules that establish good practice provide common ground. Good practice reflects the national and international understanding of research and training. This Code applies to scientific practice, which is understood to include research and training within IARC. The Code is intended for the individual researcher. The term "Researcher" applies to all categories of personnel involved in planning, conducting, evaluating, archiving and dissemination of research, including staff scientists, fellows, technicians, trainees, visiting scientists, collaborators and all allied researchers that contribute to IARC missions worldwide. All are part of the IARC community.

The IARC Code for Good Scientific Practice was developed at the request of the IARC Cabinet on 21 March 2005 to ensure that instances of fabrication, falsification, plagiarism or other serious deviation from accepted practice do not occur.

# Principles

## Integrity

Integrity involves honesty and respect for what is right and proper.

## Transparency

Research should be conducted in a transparent manner, with full and contemporaneous documentation of research methods, data and funding. The aim is accountability, with all procedures and findings being verifiable. Whenever research results are communicated, they must be based on the available data.

## Impartiality

In scientific activities, the researcher heeds no other interest than the public health interest that IARC was established to serve, and is always prepared to account for his/her actions.

## Independence

Researchers operate in a context of intellectual independence, without undue restrictions, within the scope of the work of their Institutions.

# The Principles in Practice

*Setting up the project*

IARC research studies are undertaken after detailed scientific and ethical review and are aimed to be conducted to the highest standards possible, according to an agreed and comprehensive protocol:

1. The choice of and rationale for the research question must be justified on the basis of systematic literature review.
2. The study design and choice of method must be documented, and should have passed through a scientific review.
3. Authorship responsibility should be settled at the outset of the project, including provision for necessary changes as the project develops.
4. In principle, researchers involved in IARC studies are allowed to apply to any source of funding for research, provided that (1) the scope and objective of the funding, the origin of the funds and the mechanisms for their attribution, are clearly identified; and (2) the potential commissioning party does not develop activities or sustain principles that are contrary to IARC missions, e.g. the tobacco industry. Application for external funding by IARC personnel is subject to IARC administrative rules.
5. Obtaining funding for research from third parties, such as the private sector, is guided by the principles outlined in the "WHO Guidelines on working with the private sector to achieve health outcomes".

*Conducting the project*

Data management:

1. Researchers are accountable for the quality of data collection, input, processing and storage. The need for proper recording includes not only final results but also the extensive contemporaneous documentation of all steps taken in the execution of the work, through notebooks, journals of activities highlighting decisions made, progress reports, documentation of arrangements, etc.

2. Supervisors are responsible for ensuring and verifying standards of data collection, input, processing and storage by those under their responsibility.
3. Whenever possible, raw research data, frozen data files and computer programmes should be stored.
4. Material should be indexed, annotated and archived in such a way that it can be consulted and its accuracy verified with a minimum expenditure of time and effort.


Quality control and safety:

1. Quality control measures, assessment techniques and results should be presented in parallel to (and not separated from) the research findings.
2. Appropriate quality standards include the description of basic materials; such documentation should be regularly updated and archived.
3. Quality control includes proper maintenance of the equipment and the keeping of detailed logbooks reporting equipment use and maintenance operations.
4. Supervisors are personally responsible for informing and briefing their staff about risks and safety procedures relative to their work and ensuring that these procedures are followed. In particular, they have a special responsibility in making sure that adequate protective equipment is available and used. They must take into account restrictions that may apply to staff at particularly high risk, such as pregnant women.
5. Researchers are responsible for the compliance of their work with all aspects of best safety and laboratory practice. Researchers have the right to object to the performance of a particular operation or manipulation if proper individual protection is not available.
6. Strict compliance with national and international standards with respect to the use in laboratory research of substances and agents such as radioisotopes, carcinogens, solvents, pathogens and genetically modified organisms.


Intellectual respect:

1. Researchers give others room to take their own intellectual stance. This applies particularly in case of a hierarchical relationship, like the relation between a

teacher and a student or a tutor and a PhD student or supervisor and supervisee. Remaining differences of opinion may need to be resolved at a higher level in the hierarchy.
2. The choice of methods is guided by the goal of truth-finding, not by external goals such as commercial success or political influence.
3. In assessing the performance of other researchers, a researcher heeds arguments of scientific substance.
4. A researcher only defends a certain scientific viewpoint if that viewpoint is based on sufficient scientific grounds. Competing viewpoints must be acknowledged. These general principles also apply in communicating with the general public, press and media.
5. Researchers are aware of the implications of conflicts of interest. They only accept peer review assignments on the understanding that they are free of such conflicts of interest. Conflicts of interest are handled according to the relevant IARC Guidelines.
6. In participating in peer review, researchers are respectful of intellectual property and confidentiality.

Research competence and responsibility:

1. Researchers ensure that they maintain the level of expertise required to exercise their duties. They do not accept responsibility for duties for which they lack the necessary expertise. If necessary, they actively indicate the limits of their competence.
2. Researchers provide a complete and honest overview of their skills and achievements whenever a decision concerning their duties, activities or career is pending.
3. Researchers should acknowledge and learn from their mistakes. Errors should be repaired in the best way possible.
4. Researchers are co-responsible for the scientific and societal value of the research programmes, as well as of the training programmes, in which they participate. They act according to their own preferences only insofar as this is reconcilable with this responsibility.

5. Relations among researchers and with trainees:
    a. Good mentorship of students, technicians or junior staff members is essential. The responsibilities of persons involved in training and research are to be clearly defined and observed at all times.
    b. Researchers avoid personal relationships that may give rise to reasonable doubt concerning the objectivity of their decisions, or that may result in any form of coercion or exploitation of a hierarchically subordinate person.

*Concluding the project*

1. The right of scientific publication is guaranteed within the usual rule of the scientific community, and in compliance with IARC scientific management structure.
2. Researchers have the freedom and duty to publish study findings in peer-reviewed scientific publications.
3. The main author will share the content of the peer review with the co-authors and all must accept any necessary modifications in the original paper which follow from this review.
4. Where the research has important public health implications, the researchers, using appropriate channels of communication, will arrange for their dissemination to the general public.
5. Sources of external funds must be clearly acknowledged whenever results of the relevant research are publizised, particularly in all forms of primary scientific publication. Similarly, all forms of external support to any participant into a specific IARC programme must be duly acknowledged, including training fellowships or support for travel expenses.
6. Research results must not be misrepresented: all factual conclusions must be supported by data. When material research results are omitted in the final report, the selective omission must be justified, and the relevant data collected and archived.
7. The statistical methods employed must be pertinent to the data acquired.

8. Speculation spurred by results of scientific research must be presented as such, and clearly distinguished from the conclusions based on the presented results. Suggestions for follow-up research may rest on speculation, in the form of an interpretation of the acquired results.
9. Credit is awarded where credit is deserved, through authorship or acknowledgment and through accurate sourcing of references.
10. Every researcher is entitled to authorship, irrespective of the category of staff. This also applies to trainees and IARC visiting scientists. In acknowledging authorship, rules common to the scientific discipline are observed. Authorship implies a substantial contribution to design, planning, supervision or conduct of research, as well as to data analysis, interpretation or preparation for publication. Contributions of a strictly logistical nature are usually acknowledged by a footnote in the relevant section of the publication. Nevertheless, technical contributions of particular merit or reflecting a high level of expertise may be credited by authorship.
11. Accurate sourcing of references is practised in any publication. References are sourced independently of their publication language, of their country of origin, or of the impact factor of the journal in which they are published. This also applies to information gathered via the Internet.

*Following publication of a project*

The corresponding author is responsible for management of correspondence (private or published) that may follow from the publication of the project, and all the authors should be kept informed of these developments.

Since the objective of IARC is to promote international collaboration in cancer research, requests for use of the data on which the project is founded should be encouraged, with due regard to the terms on which the data were obtained and stipulations that may have been made in connection with the project at the stage it was ethically reviewed.

## Concluding remarks

This Code exists to promote the highest standards of research conduct for the IARC community and is based on integrity, transparency, impartiality and independence.

## Acknowledgements

In the preparation of this Code we have studied a number of documents which have greatly assisted us in formulating this proposal. We also have taken into account comments on the draft document from IARC collaborators. We would like to thank all that have contributed to the revisions.

# Appendices

This appendix lists a selection from the documents that we studied in the development of this code, to illustrate the literature it is derived from and draw attention to these particularly relevant documents.

- IARC Statute, Rules and Regulations (http://www.iarc.fr/en/About-IARC/Governance/IARC-Statute-Rules-and-Regulations-Twelfth-Edition-2003)
- Standard of Conduct for the International Civil Service (2004) (http://icsc.un.org/resources/pdfs/general/standardsE.pdf)
- WHO Guidelines on working with the private sector to achieve health outcomes (http://ftp.who.int/gb/archive/pdf_files/EB107/ee20.pdf)
- WHO Whistleblower Protection: Policy and Procedures, November 2006 (WHO Information Note 44/2006)
- IARC Safety Manual
- IARC Notebooks Instructions
- WHO Performance Management and Development System
- IARC Guidelines on Ethics (http://ethics.iarc.fr/index.php)
- European Commission Recommendation of 11 March 2005 on the European Charter for Researchers and on a Code of Conduct for the Recruitment of Researchers (http://ec.europa.eu/eracareers/pdf/am509774CEE_EN_E4.pdf)
- Executive Order N° 668 of 28 June 2005 on the Danish Committees on Scientific Dishonesty (http://fi.dk/portal/pls/pr05/docs/1/1134036.PDF)
- Official Norwegian Report NOU 2005:1 – Good Research, Better Health (http://www.helsetilsynet.no/upload/english/nou_2005_1_english%20summary.pdf)
- Council of Science Editors' White Paper on Promoting Integrity in Scientific Journal Publications (http://www.councilscienceeditors.org/editorial_policies/whitepaper/entire_whitepaper.pdf)
- International Committee of Medical Journal Editors' Uniform Requirements for Manuscripts Submitted to Biomedical Journals: Writing and Editing for Biomedical Publication, February 2006 (http://www.icmje.org/)